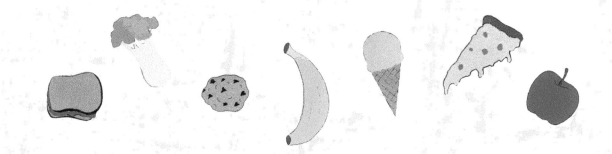

WAS IT SOMETHING I ATE?

the type 1 diabetes myth buster for kids

Written and illustrated
by
Amelia Pinegar

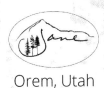

Orem, Utah

For Ralph,
who believed in the idea.

For Melissa,
who believed in the artist.

For Mom and Dad,
who have always believed in the writer.

And for all my friends with T1D.

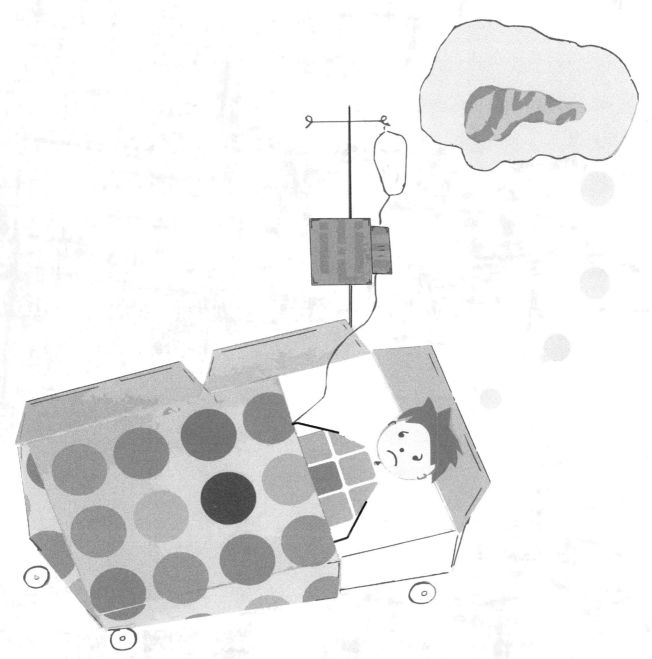

I'm lying here in my hospital bed
with thoughts of my pancreas stuck in my head.

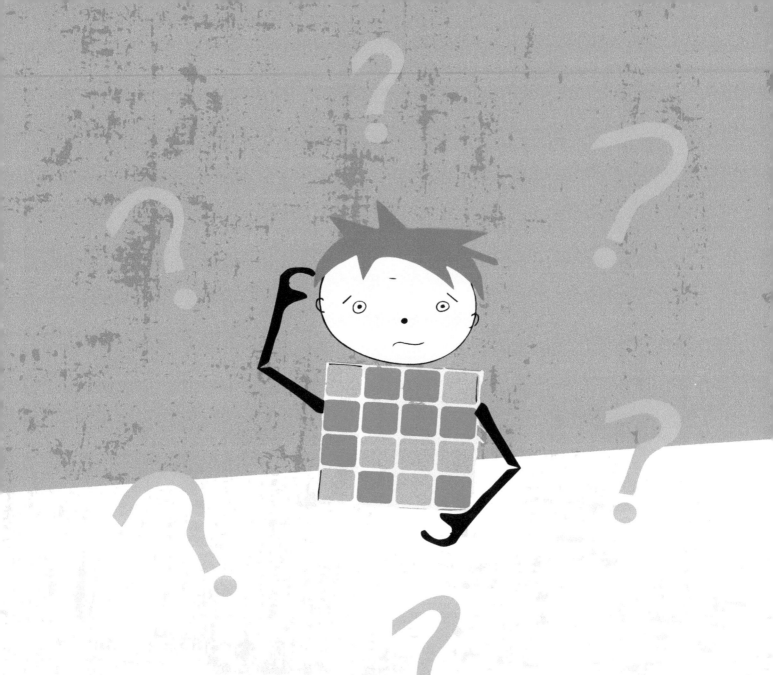

Pancreas, pancreas, what does that mean?
It's something inside me that I've never seen.

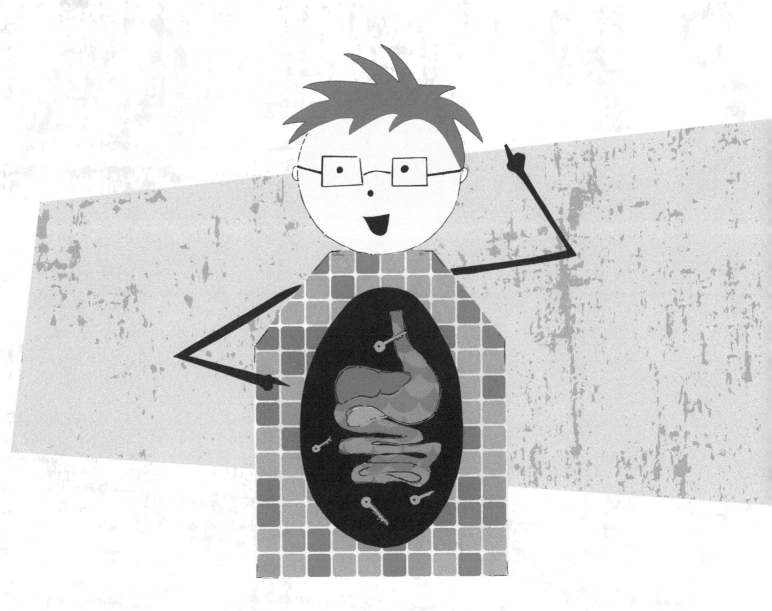

It's s'posed to make insulin—a magic key—
that opens up doors on the inside of me.
With doors open wide, that key is my tool.
Insulin helps me turn food into fuel!

But my keys are lost—they're no help when I eat.
Now the blood inside me is getting too sweet.

"Diabetes," they say, "is what happens now."
But could somebody please explain to me HOW?

HOW did this happen? And WHY am I here?
WHAT's the next step? Is this something to fear?

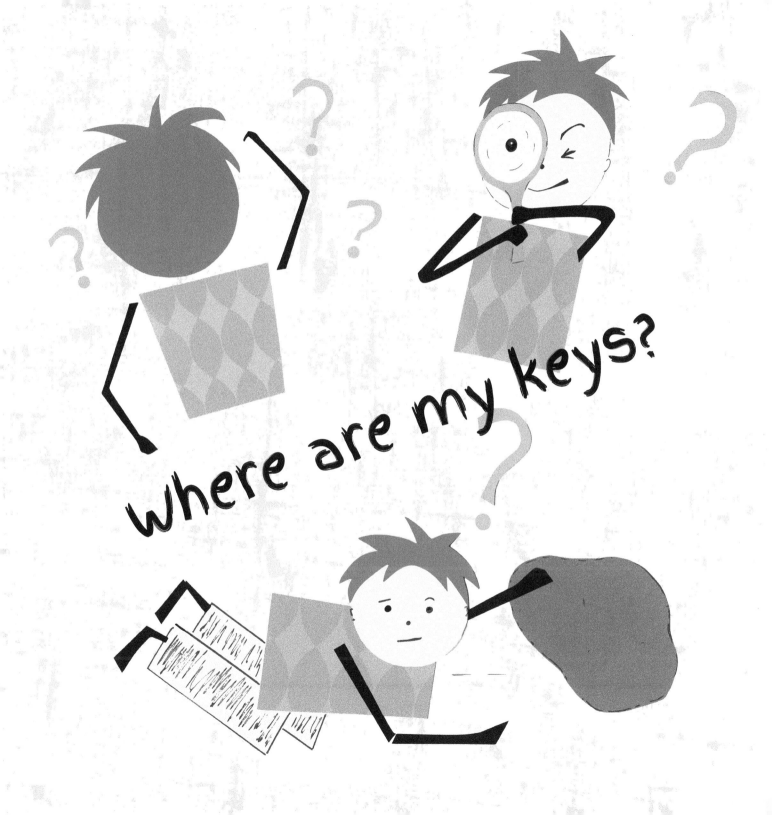

They call it an autoimmune disease.
But ah-ah-ACHOO! That word makes me sneeze!

I look to my nurse to help me find out,
"exactly WHAT are they talking about?!"

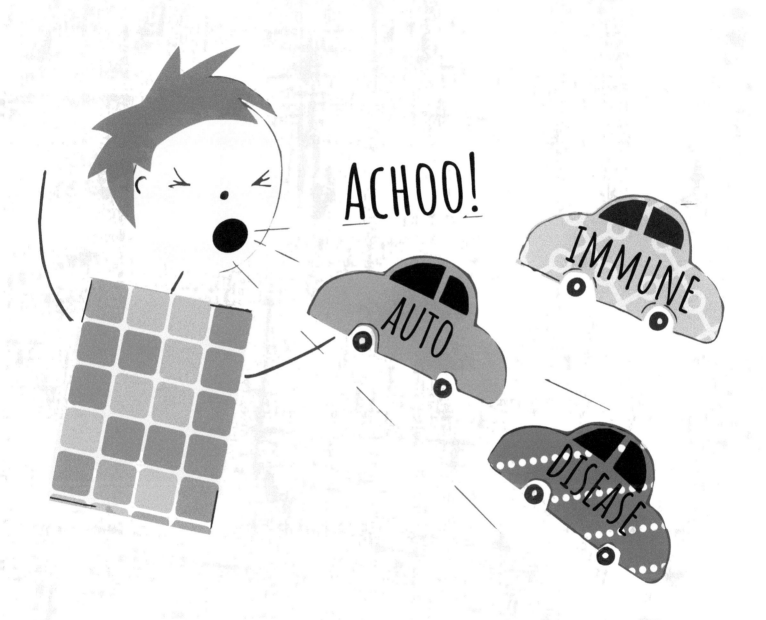

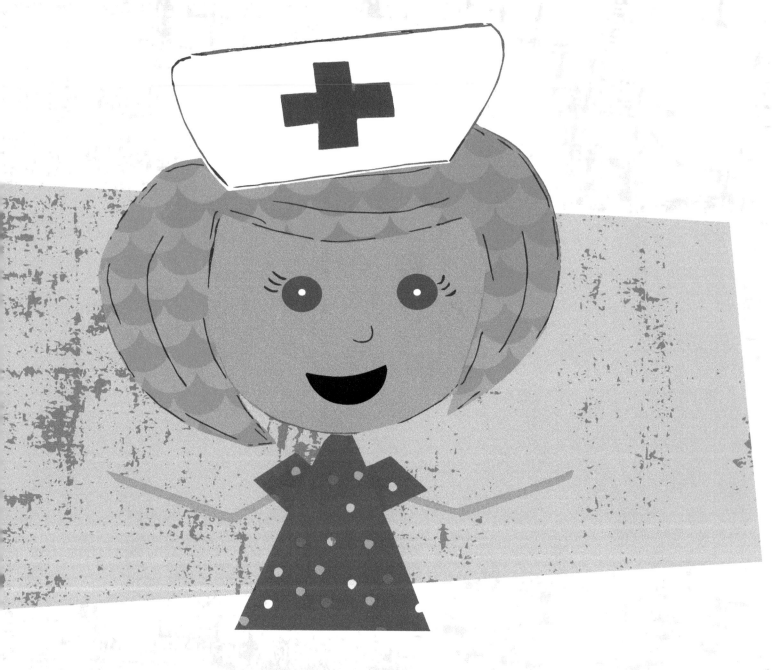

"Auto is simply a word that means self.
Your body is fighting against your own health."

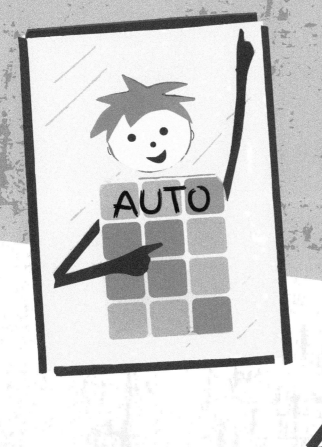
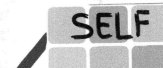

A fight inside me seems kinda outrageous.
So I ask my nurse, "is this thing contagious?"

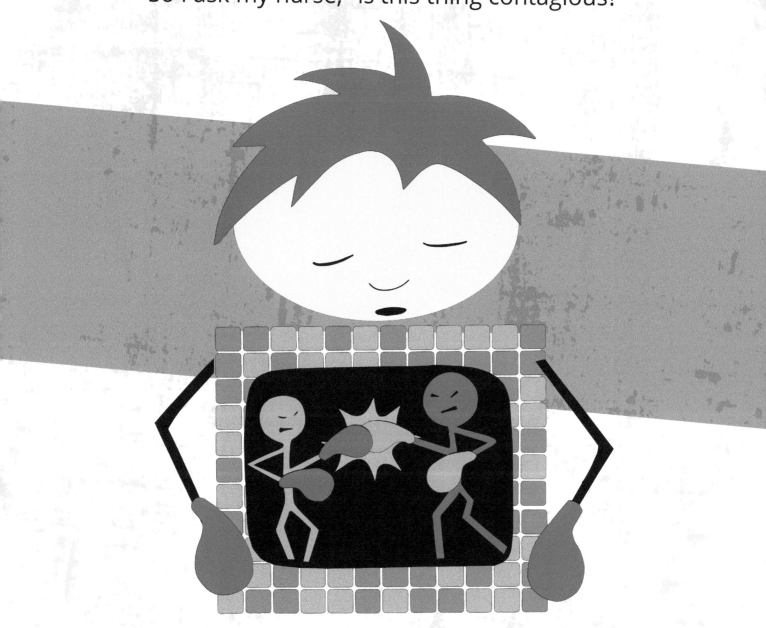

She shakes her head no. "This is not like the flu.
No one else will get sick from being with you."

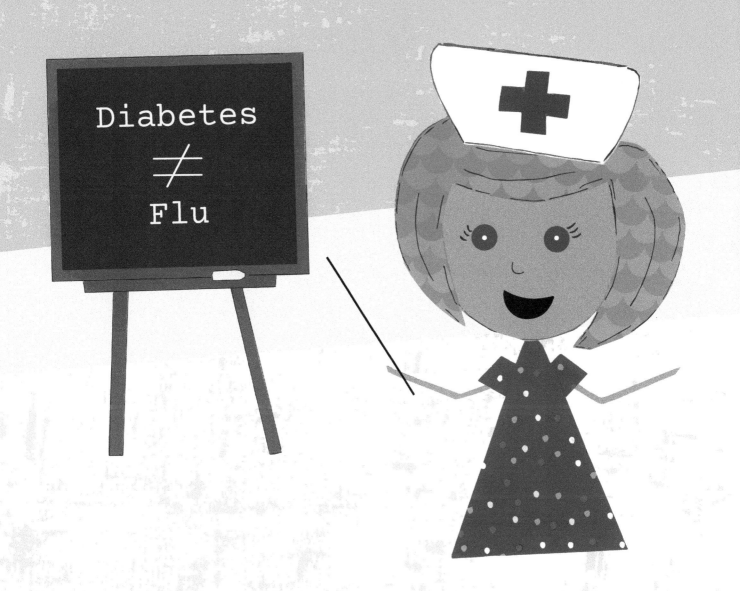

"Buuuut.....
Without that insulin, your blood sugar soars—
up the wall, through the roof, and right out the door.

That high blood sugar can make you so sick.
You need insulin and you need it quick!

So we'll give you shots to help you get better..."

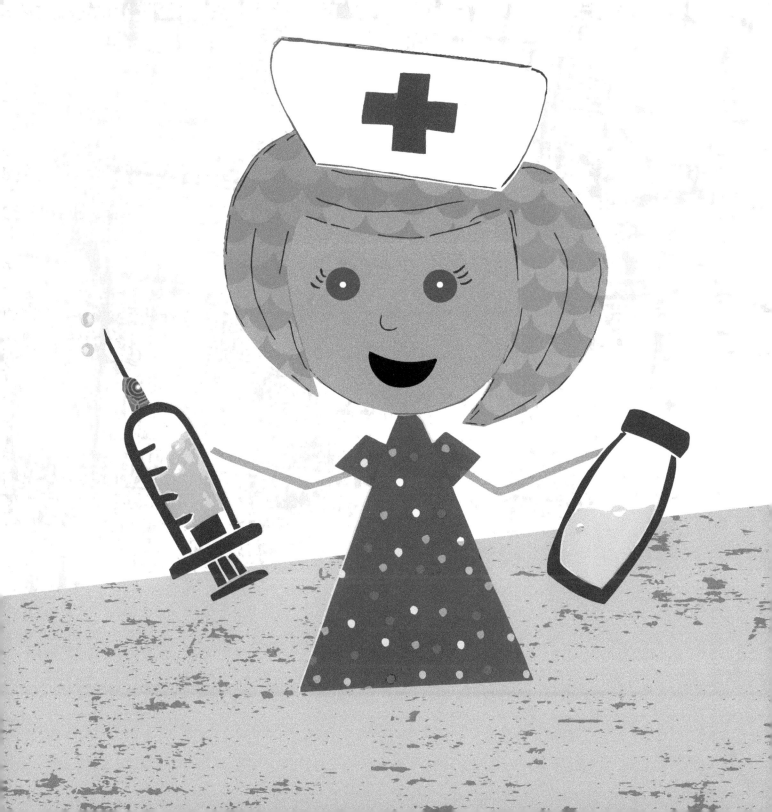

"In no time flat,

you'll be

OVER

the

weather."

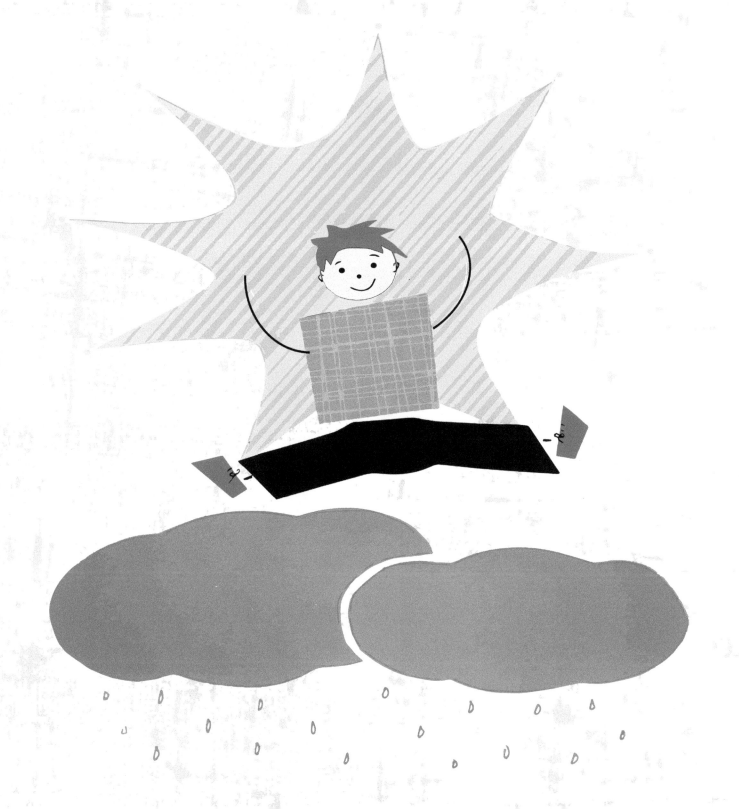

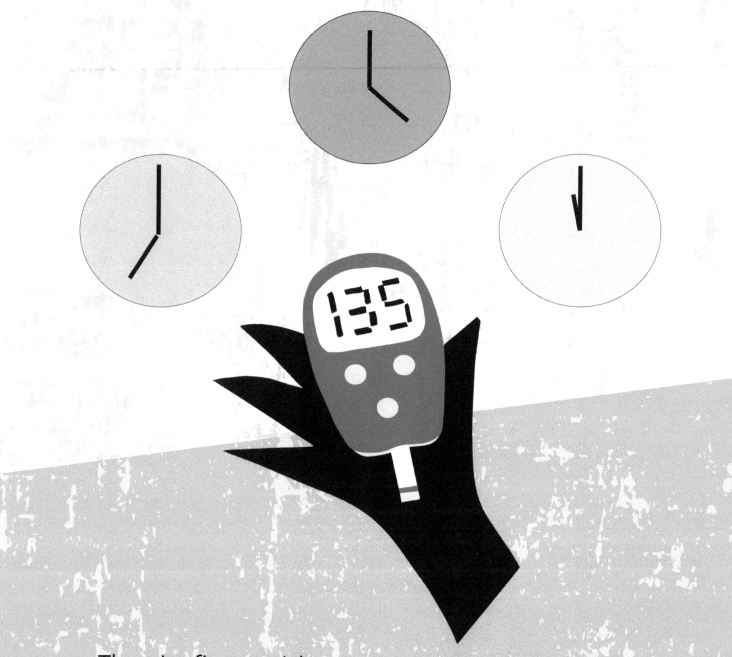

There're finger sticks, meters, and testing a bunch.
They happen at breakfast, and dinner, AND lunch!

I feel like a porcupine lives in this bed.
I'd rather play baseball with Grandpa instead.

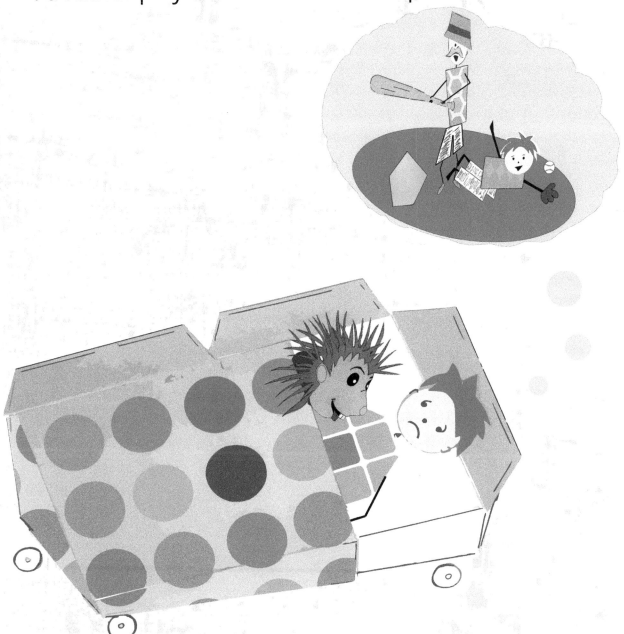

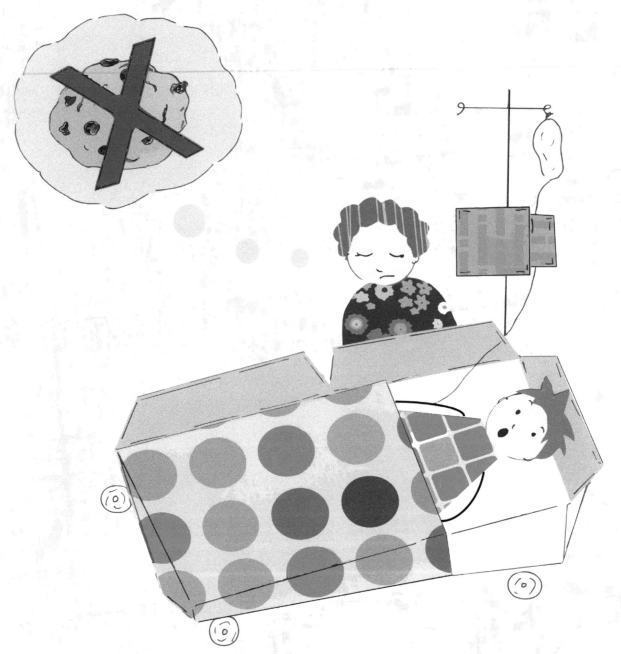

Grandma Crumb sits beside me, wearing a frown.
"No more cookies for you," she says, looking down.

What? No more cookies? What a terrible fate!
"Jumping jellybeans! Was it something I ate?!"

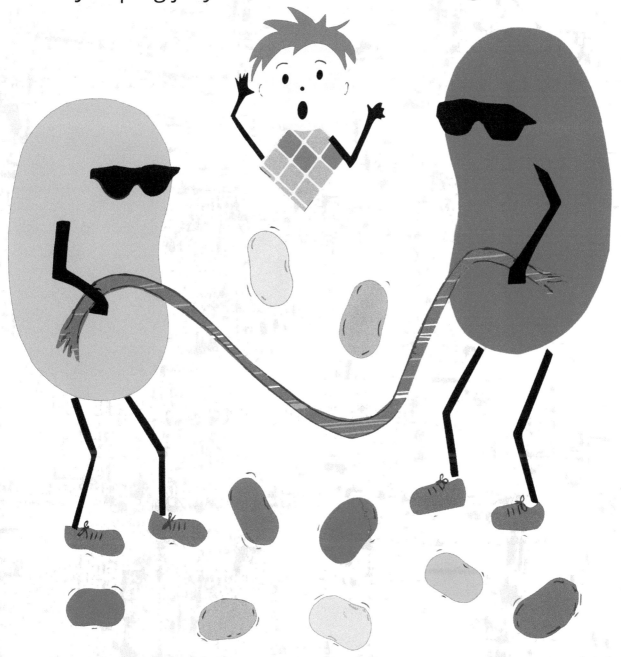

My nurse overhears and says with a smile,
"That's a tall tale that goes on for a mile."

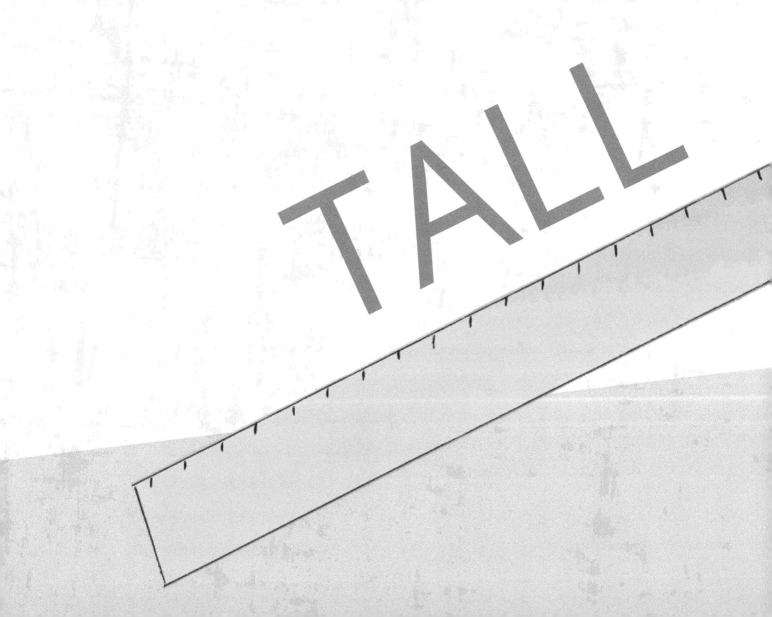

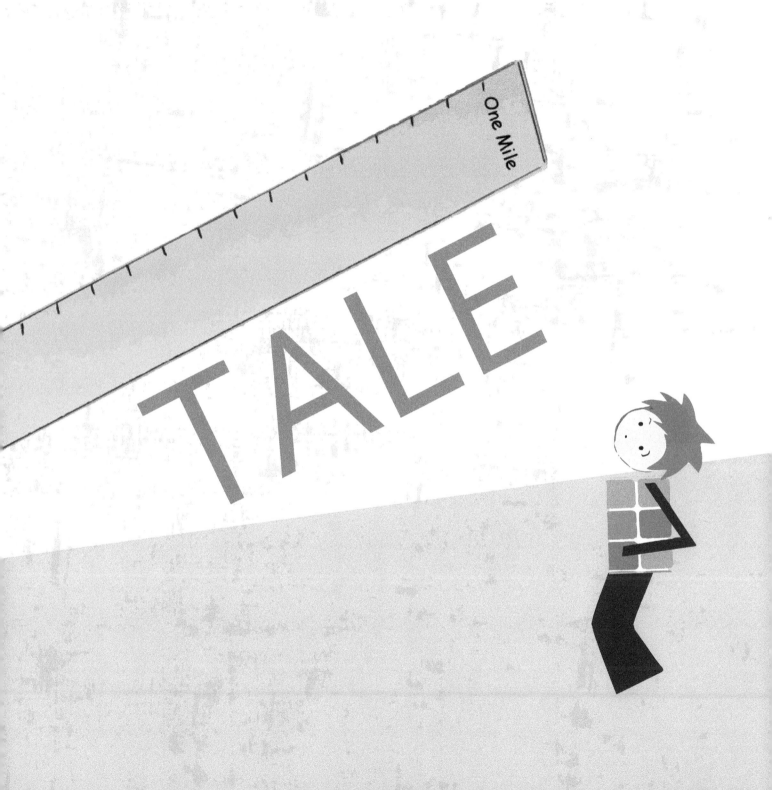

"It was nothing you ate that caused this disease.
You can still eat cookies, if that's what you please.

Of course, you'll want veggies and healthy foods too.
They'll give you the strength to do all that you do."

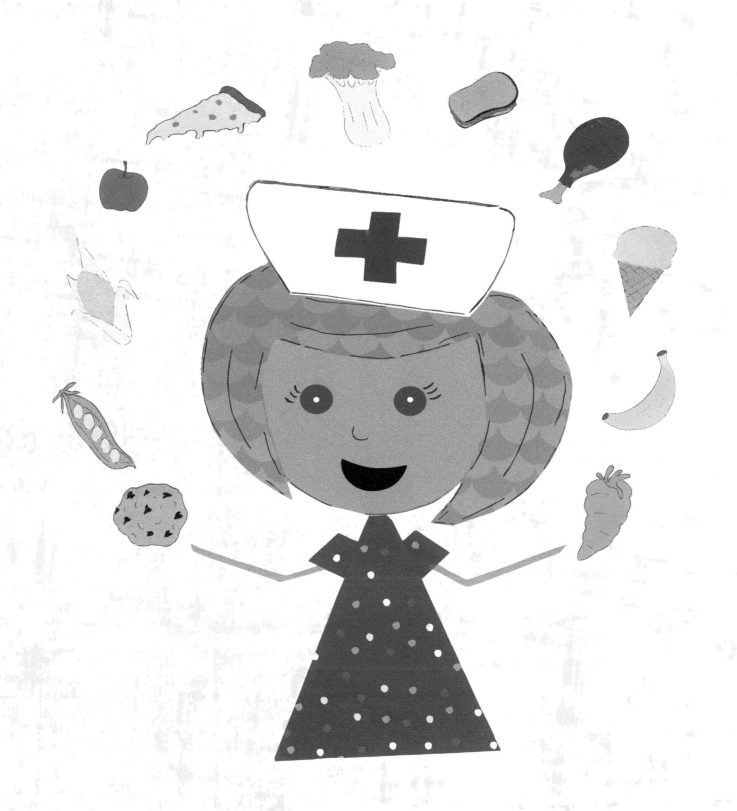

"No, this wasn't your food by any old means.
It had more to do with the state of your genes."

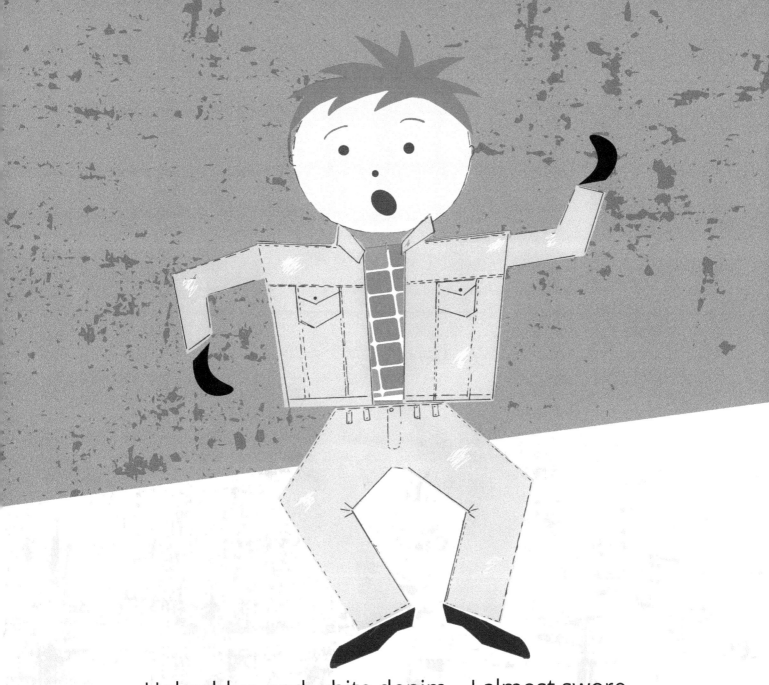

Holey blue and white denim—I almost swore.
"You mean to tell me it was something I wore?!"

"It's genes with a G, not jeans with a J!
They're the ones that code for your D-N-A.
The D-N-A is your building chart.
It helps your body to grow each part."

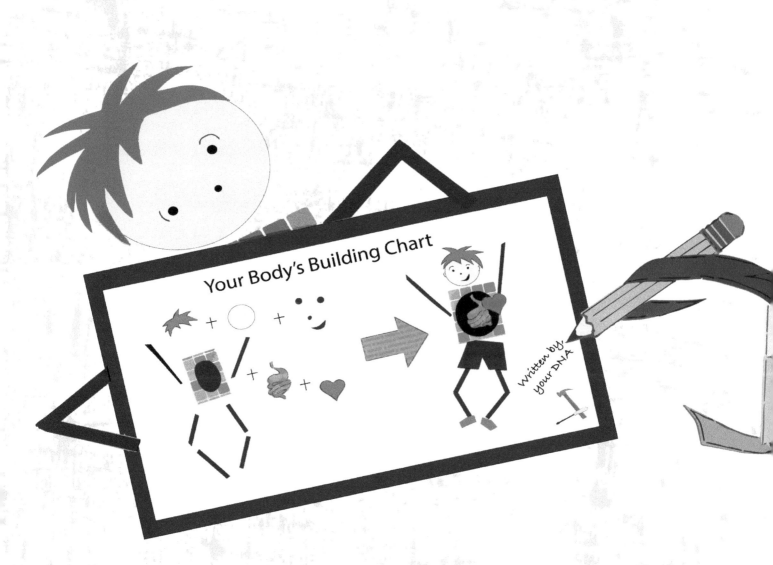

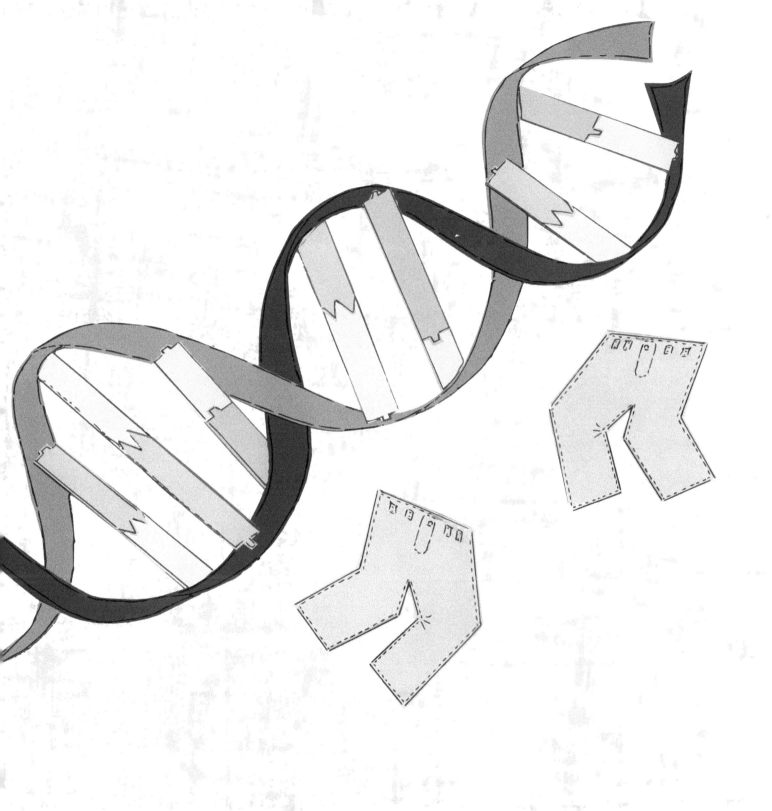

"What dumb, rotten luck," I say with a scowl.
Then the nurse turns back like a wise old owl.

"It's fine to feel sad—but don't let it stay.
Don't let diabetes get in your way..."

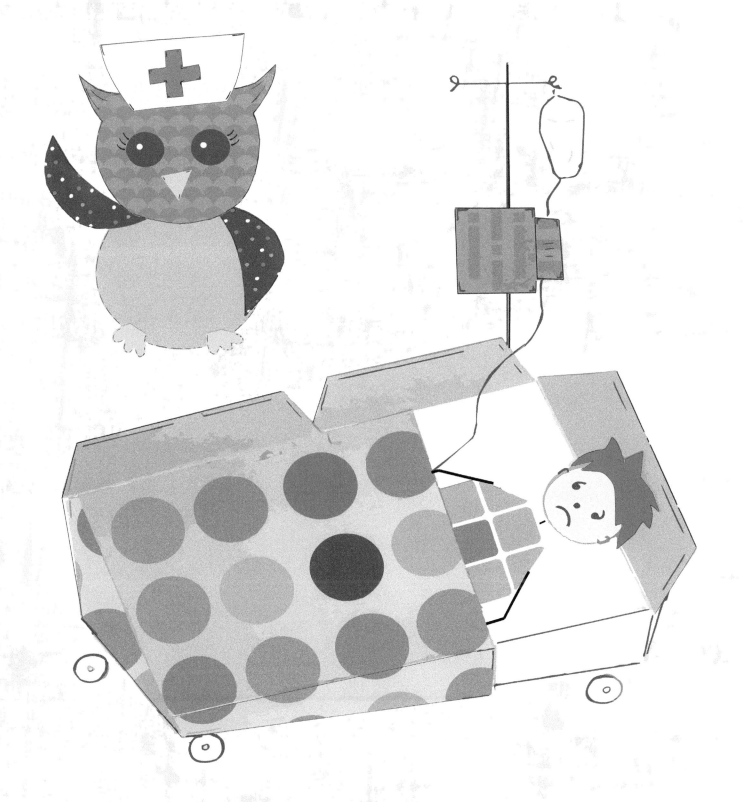

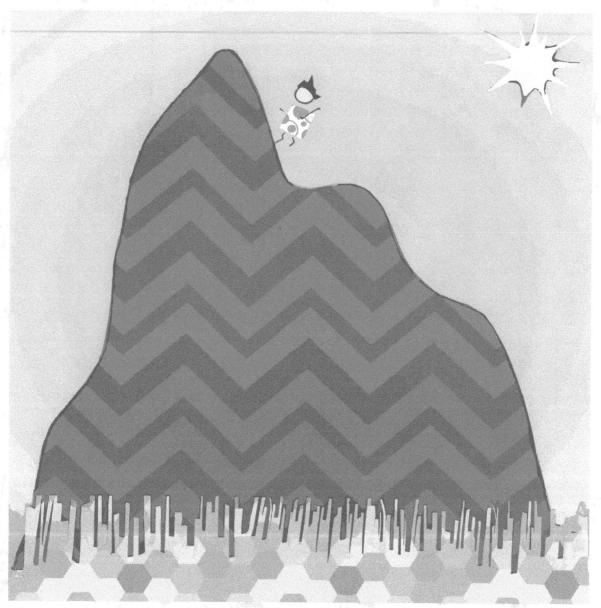

"...of laughing, and living, and doing a lot,
of climbing great mountains right up to the top."

"Travel the world. Write a best-selling book.
Try out for the play and learn how to cook."

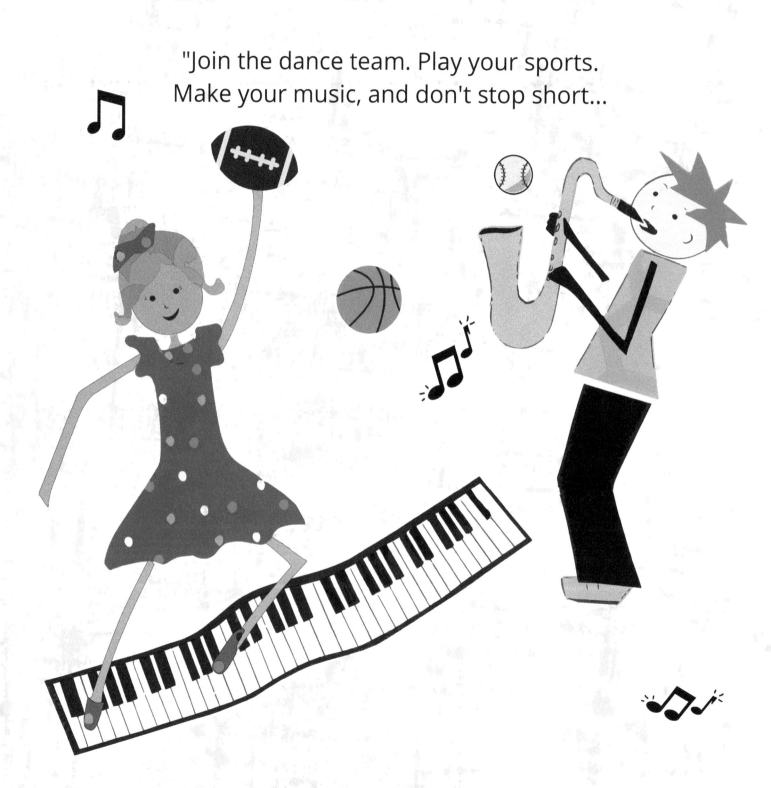

"Join the dance team. Play your sports.
Make your music, and don't stop short...

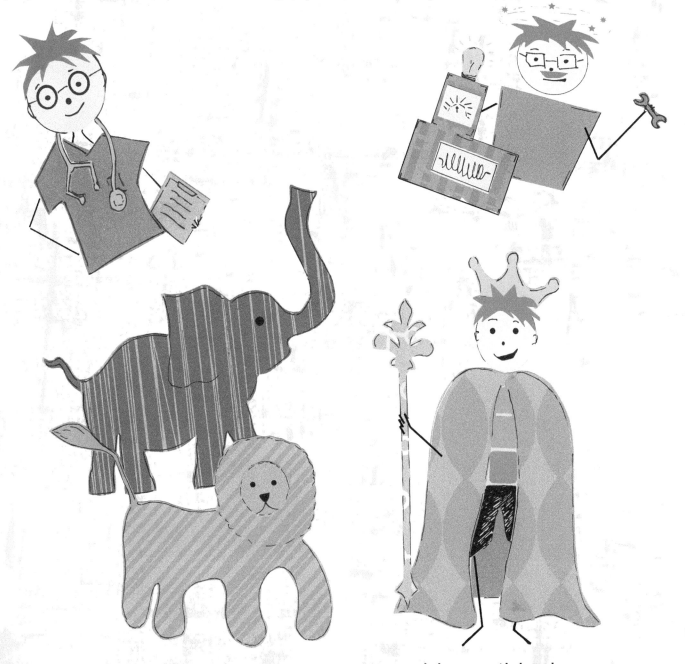

...of all the great dreams you could possibly dream.
Be a doctor, inventor, or zookeeper king."

"Diabetes is just a curve ball at bat.
And I'm pretty sure that YOU can beat that!"

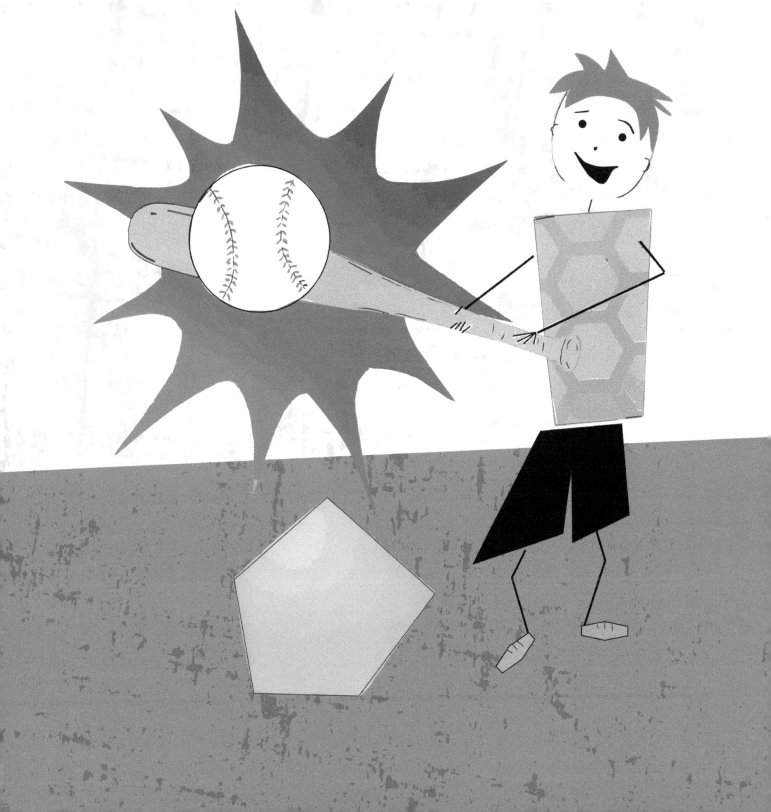

Use this page to draw a picture of what you want to be when you grow up.

Autoimmune disease (ah-toe-ih-mune dih-zeeze):

a disease where the body attacks part of itself because it doesn't recognize that part.

Diabetes (die-uh-bee-tees):

an autoimmune disease that attacks the pancreas so that it no longer makes insulin.

Hyperglycemia (hi-per-gly-see-me-uh):

high blood sugar (hyper means high). Signs of high blood sugar include drinking a lot, peeing a lot, feeling hungry, tired, grumpy, and sick to your stomach.

Hypoglycemia (hi-po-gly-see-me-uh):

low blood sugar (hypo means low). Signs of low blood sugar include feeling shaky, weak, dizzy, hungry, confused, and sweaty.

Insulin (in-suh-lin):

the tool your body uses to help move sugar from your bloodstream into your body's cells to be used as fuel.

Pancreas (pan-cree-us):

the part of your body that makes insulin.

Amelia Pinegar (rhymes with vinegar) enjoys reading, writing, and hiking the Utah mountain trails. She currently works as a diabetes educator and is studying to become a nurse practitioner. She wholeheartedly wishes more textbooks were written in rhyme.

Book Design by Melissa Cox

ISBN 9781735644028

10 9 8 7 6 5 4 3 2 1

The art for this book was created by hand using paper, scissors, glue, and all of the best kindergarten memories.

⧉ @storybookjane

CPSIA information can be obtained
at www.ICGtesting.com
Printed in the USA
LVHW070019260821
696087LV00008B/996